Go Safe

• Press out stickers.
• Lick and stick.

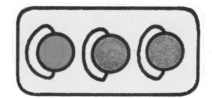

Ask an adult to remove the poster in the center of the book. Carefully open staples; lift out poster and unfold it. Close staples to keep book intact.

Use the stickers for the poster, inside pages or wherever you would like.

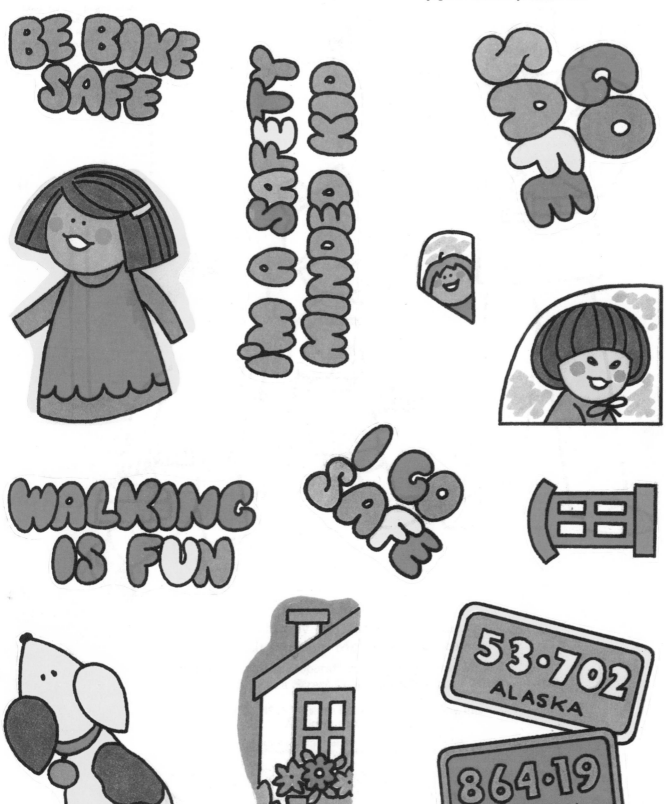

Walk Safe

It is always best to walk on the sidewalk. But if you must walk along the road, always walk on the left side, facing traffic. Walk close to the edge and try to walk with an adult or older friend.

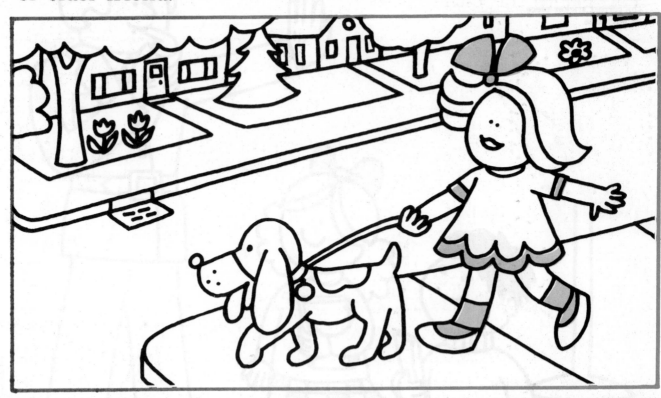

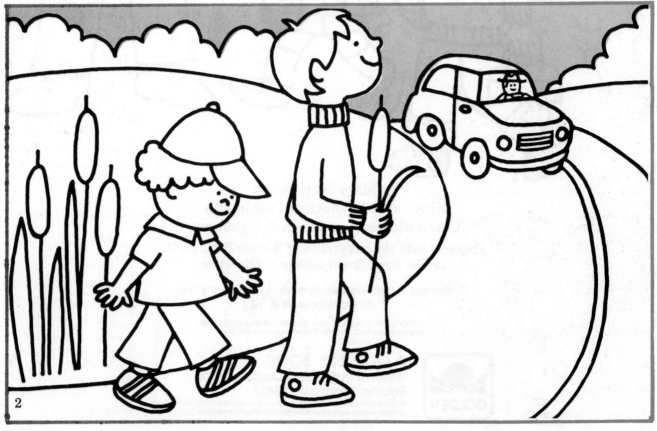

Stay in the Crosswalk

Walk in the crosswalk when crossing the street. The crosswalk is at the corner. Never cross between parked cars. Help these children cross each street correctly, so they can get to the park.

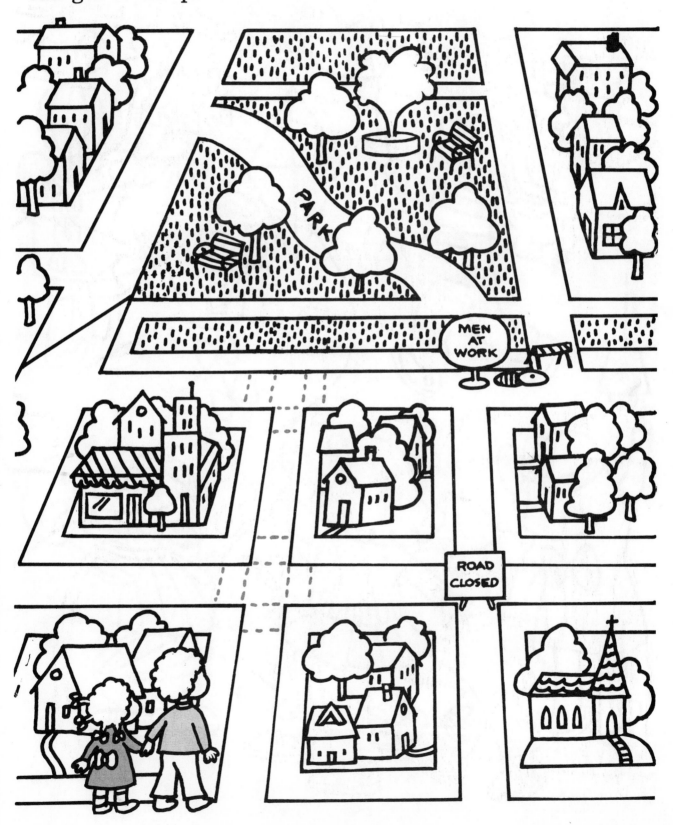

Left Is Left

Do you know which is your left hand? Look at the children on these two pages. Draw a circle around each child using his or her left hand. Draw an X through pictures of children using their right hands.

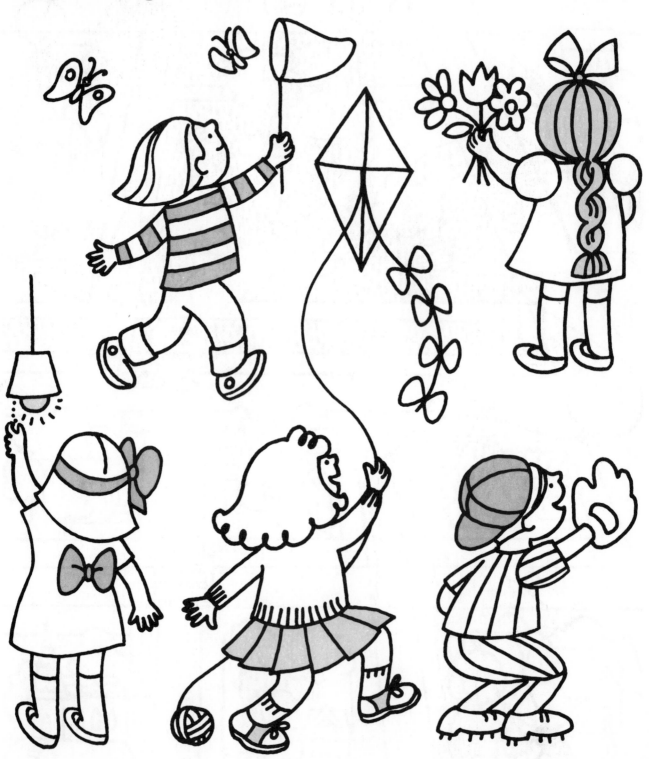

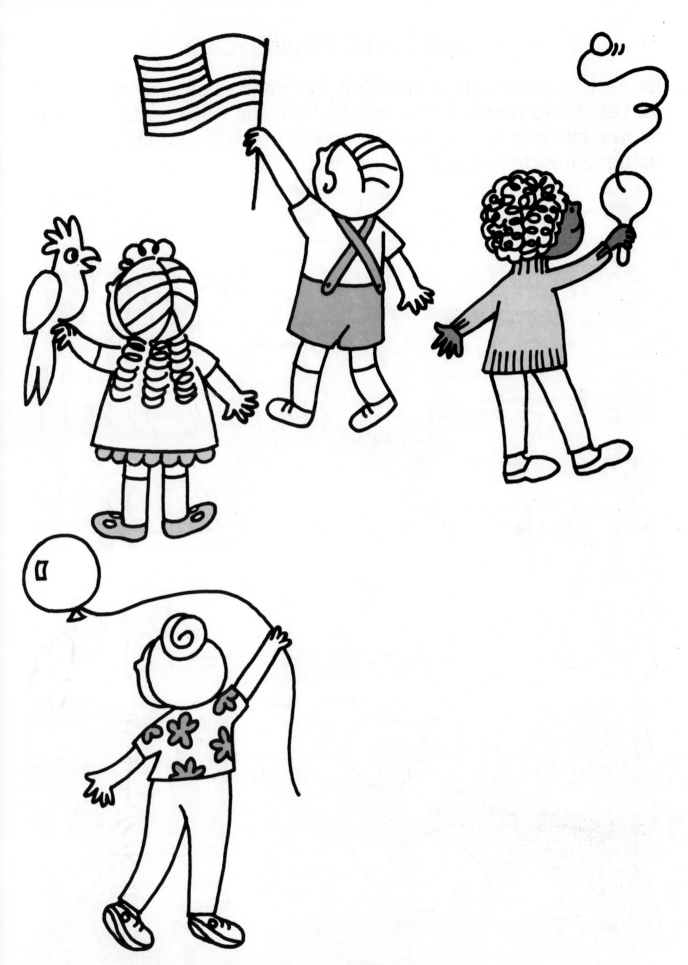

Trace your left hand with a pencil or crayon.

Look Left, Right, Left

Look left, look right, then look left again before crossing the street. If you are with an adult, hold his or her hand when crossing. Look for all kinds of vehicles before crossing. See how many vehicles you can find in this puzzle. Circle words across, up and down. Use the picture clues to help you.

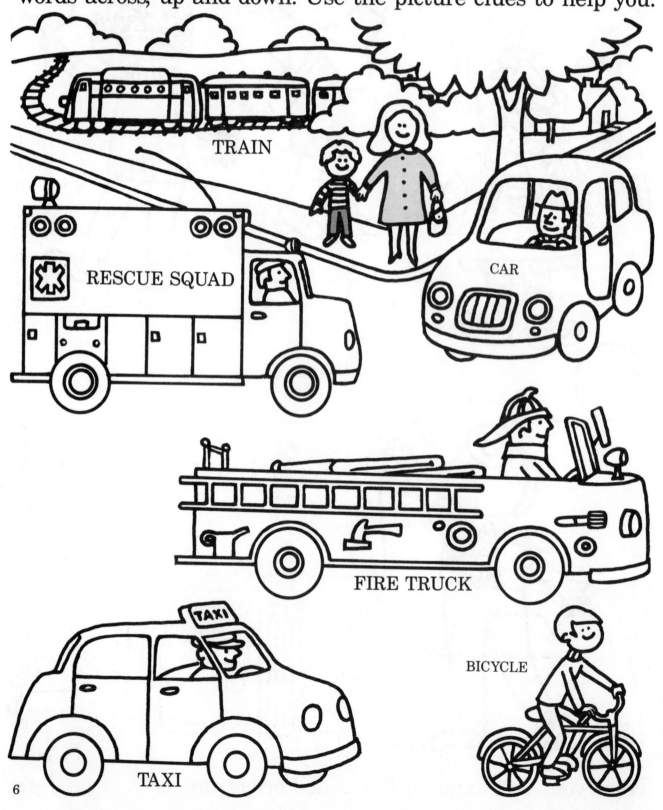

TRAIN

RESCUE SQUAD

CAR

FIRE TRUCK

BICYCLE

TAXI

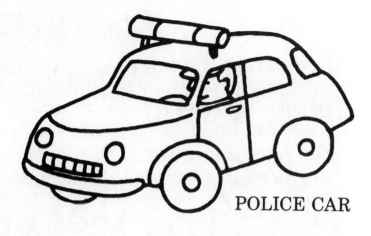

POLICE CAR

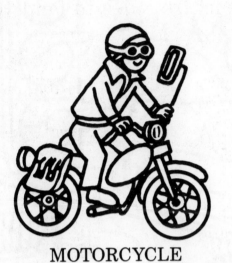

MOTORCYCLE

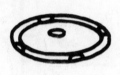

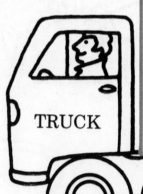

TRUCK

```
V  M  O  T  O  R  C  Y  C  L  E
E  P  T  O  L  E  V  B  G  C  K
H  O  M  T  K  S  L  N  T  Z  K
I  L  Y  R  G  H  R  T  R  Z  K
C  I  T  A  B  U  E  U  B  T  U
R  C  B  I  N  E  L  C  K  R  C
G  A  G  N  G  S  G  Y  C  O  R
N  R  X  C  I  Q  R  C  C  A  T
T  O  Q  I  L  U  T  I  A  G  I
O  F  U  R  S  H  D  F  B  B  F
```

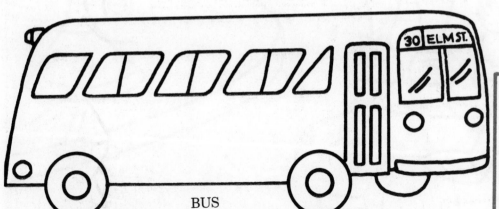

BUS

7

Obey Traffic Lights

If you cross the street where there is a special light for pedestrians (someone who walks), cross when the light shows GREEN or WALK.

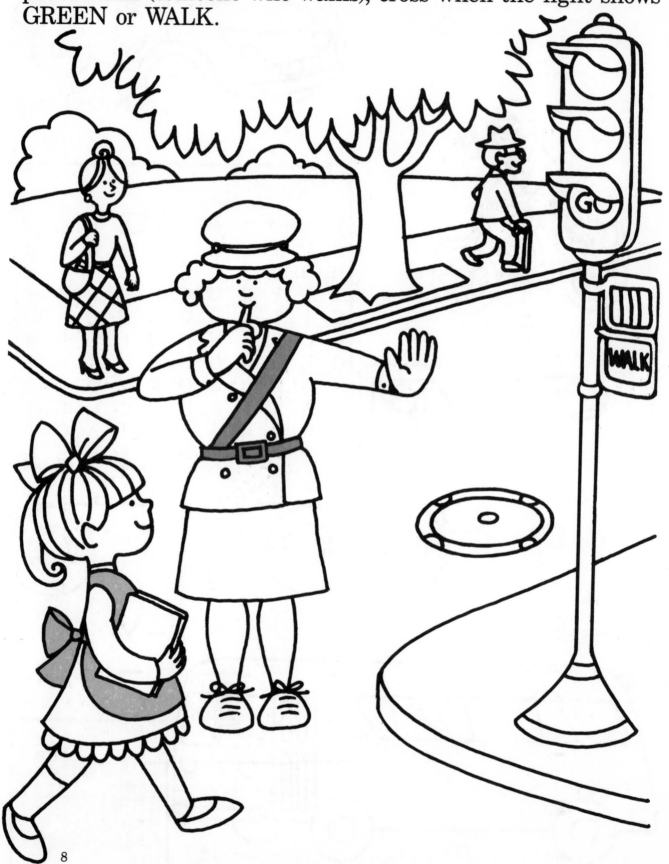

Red Light/Green Light

Do you know where the green light is on the traffic light?
Follow the color by number code to complete this light.

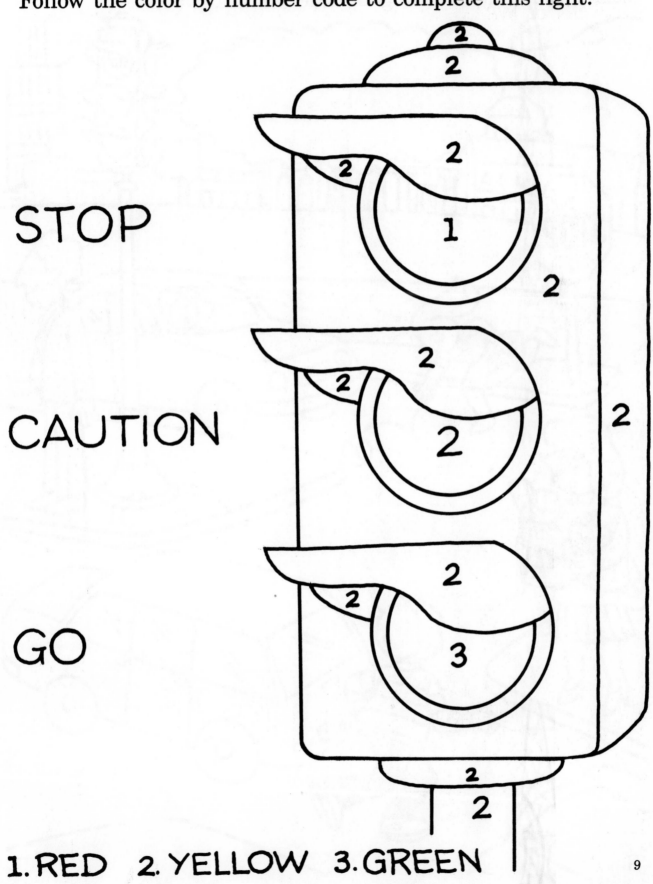

STOP

CAUTION

GO

1. RED   2. YELLOW   3. GREEN

What's Unsafe?

Draw an X through all of the things that are unsafe in this scene. Remember your good safety rules.

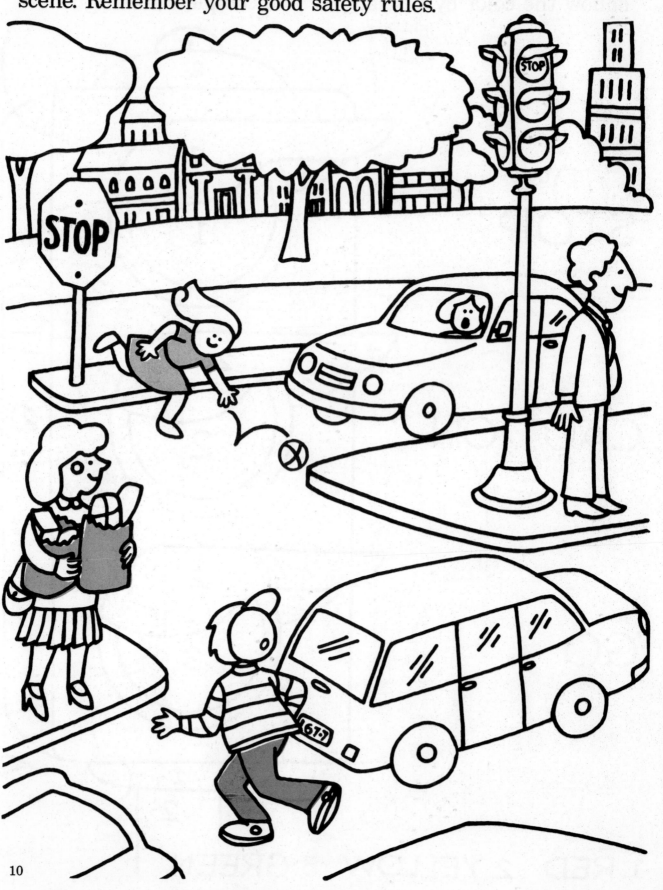

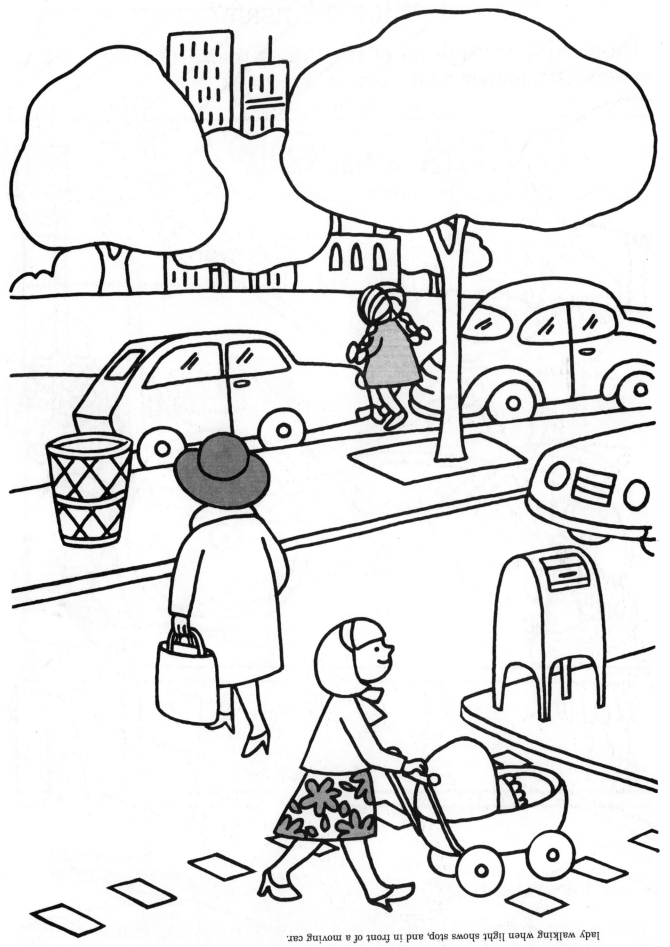

Answers: girl chasing ball, boy running between moving cars, girl walking between parked cars, lady walking when light shows stop, and in front of a moving car.

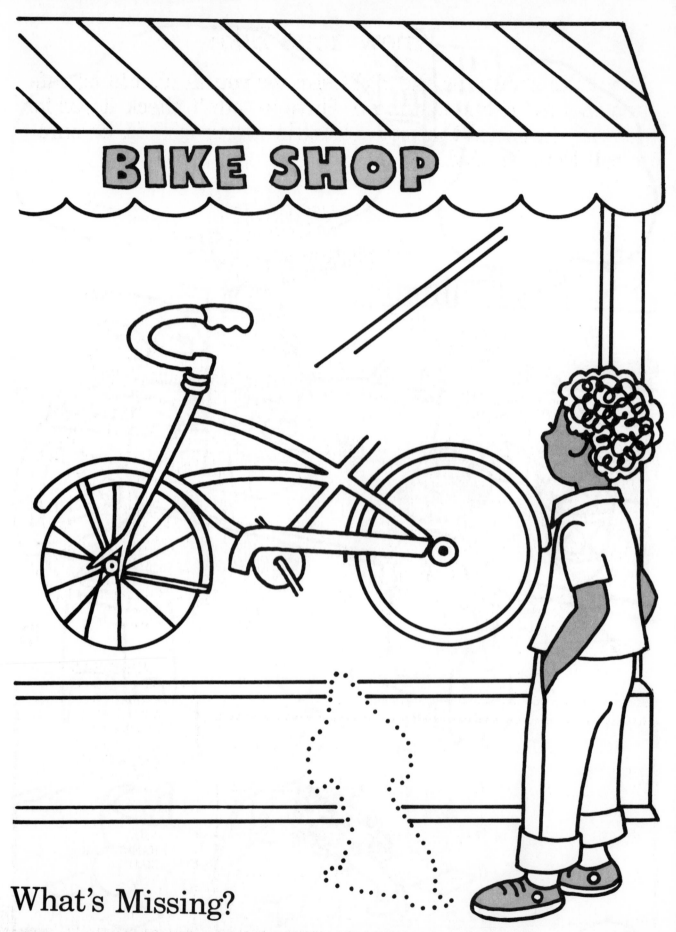

What's Missing?

When you get your first bike it is very exciting. Some things are missing from this bike. Can you draw them in?

Know Your Bike

Your bike should be the right size for you. It should be safe and in good riding condition. Have an adult check it out for you. If you notice that something is wrong with it, be sure to tell Mom or Dad.

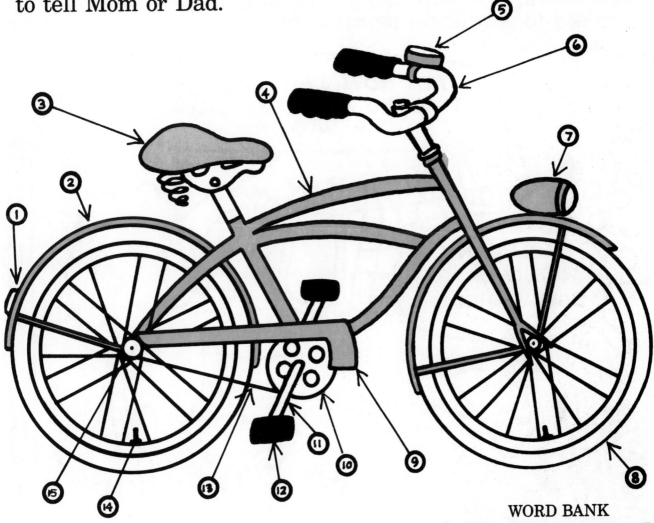

Use the word bank to help you label this bike.

1. _____

2. _____

3. _____

4. _____

5. _____

6. _____

7. _____

8. _____

9. _____

10. _____

11. _____

12. _____

13. _____

14. _____

15. _____

WORD BANK

SADDLE
BELL
CHAIN GUARD
REAR REFLECTOR
CHAIN WHEEL
FENDER
CRANK
BRAKE
LIGHT
TIRE
HANDLEBAR
CHAIN
PEDAL
TIRE VALVE
FRAME

Stay Close to Home

It is a good idea to ride your bike close to your home. That way Mom, Dad or the person taking care of you can see you and always know where you are. If you are outside alone while riding your bike, <u>never</u> ride away from where you are supposed to be without permission!

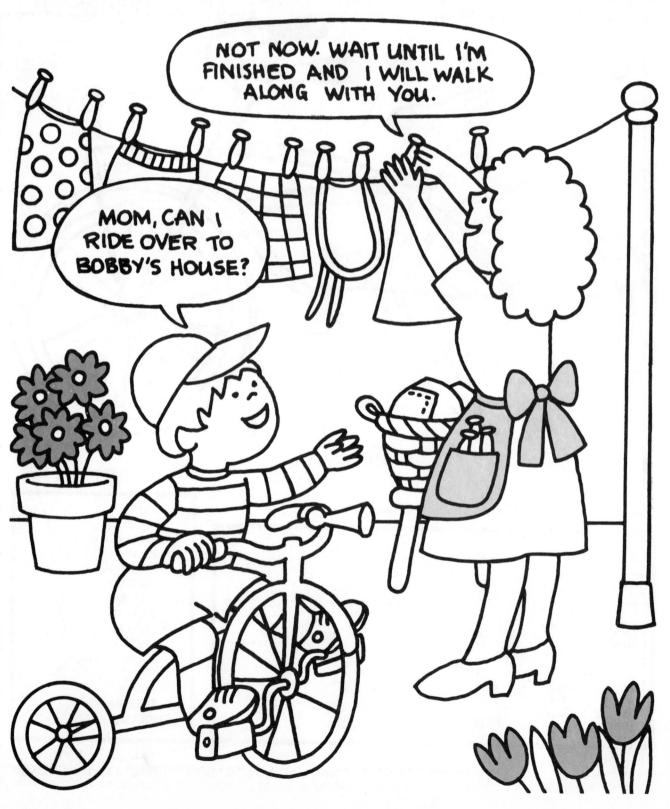

Riding too far away from home can cause you some problems! You may get lost or confused about where you are. Johnny didn't ask permission to ride to his friend's house and now he is lost. Can you take him safely back to his home?

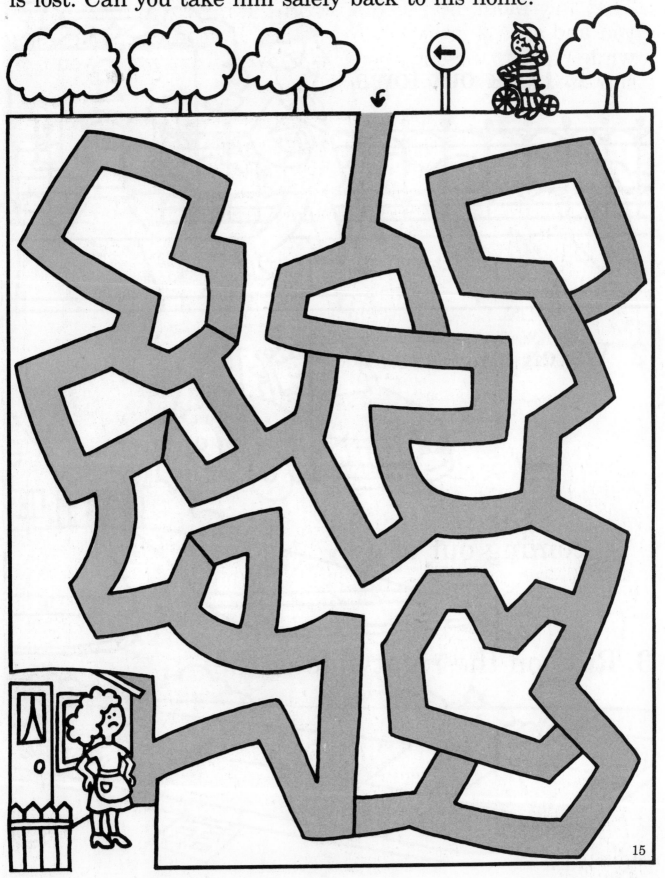

Sidewalk Riders

If you ride your bike on the sidewalk, learn the rules below.
Use the pictures to help you read each sentence.

1. Look out for a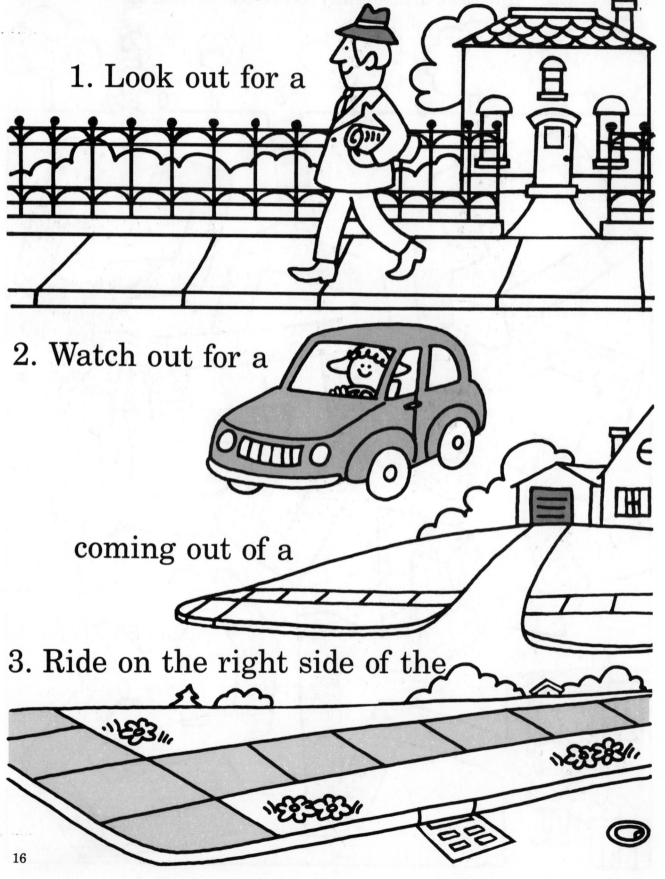

2. Watch out for a

   coming out of a

3. Ride on the right side of the

4. Look out for 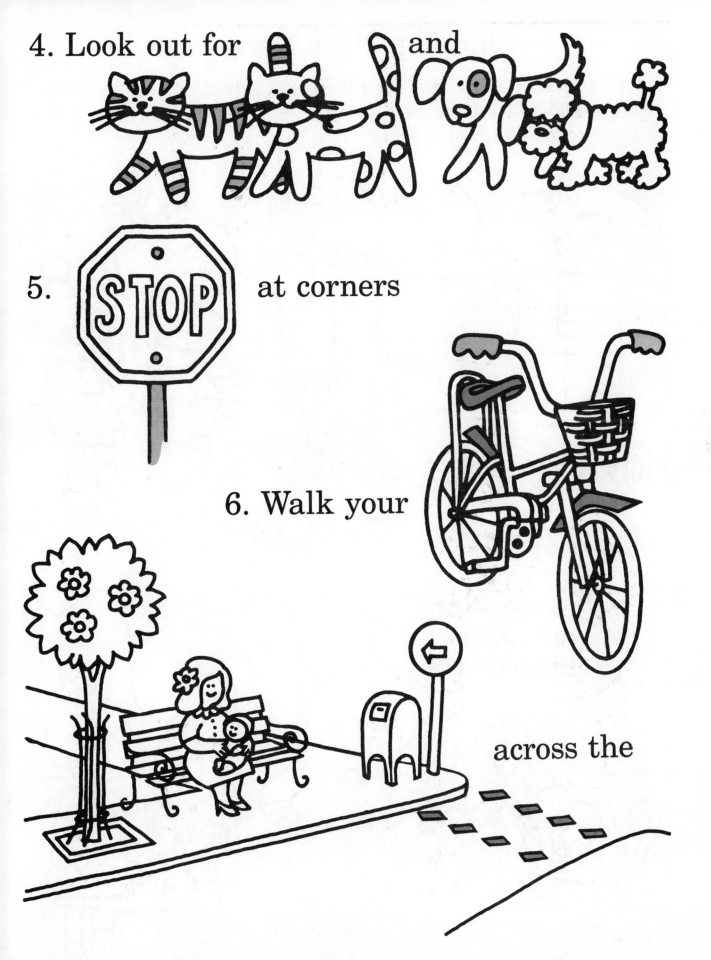 and

5. STOP at corners

6. Walk your

across the

Showing Off Is Dangerous

Stunts or tricks are not for biking on streets or sidewalks. Keep your feet on the pedals and both hands on the handlebars, except when signaling.

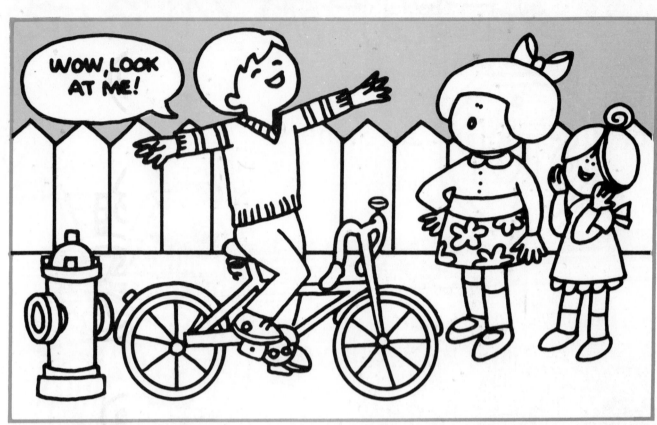

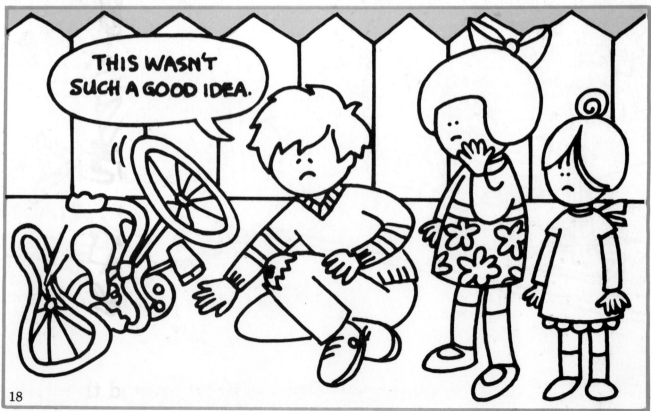

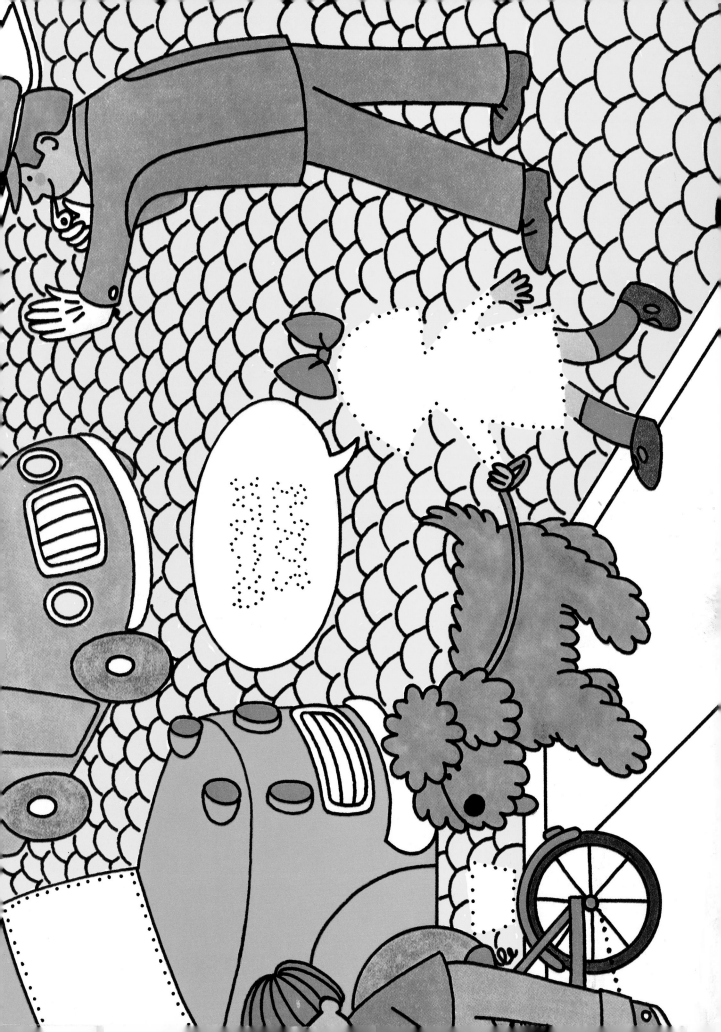

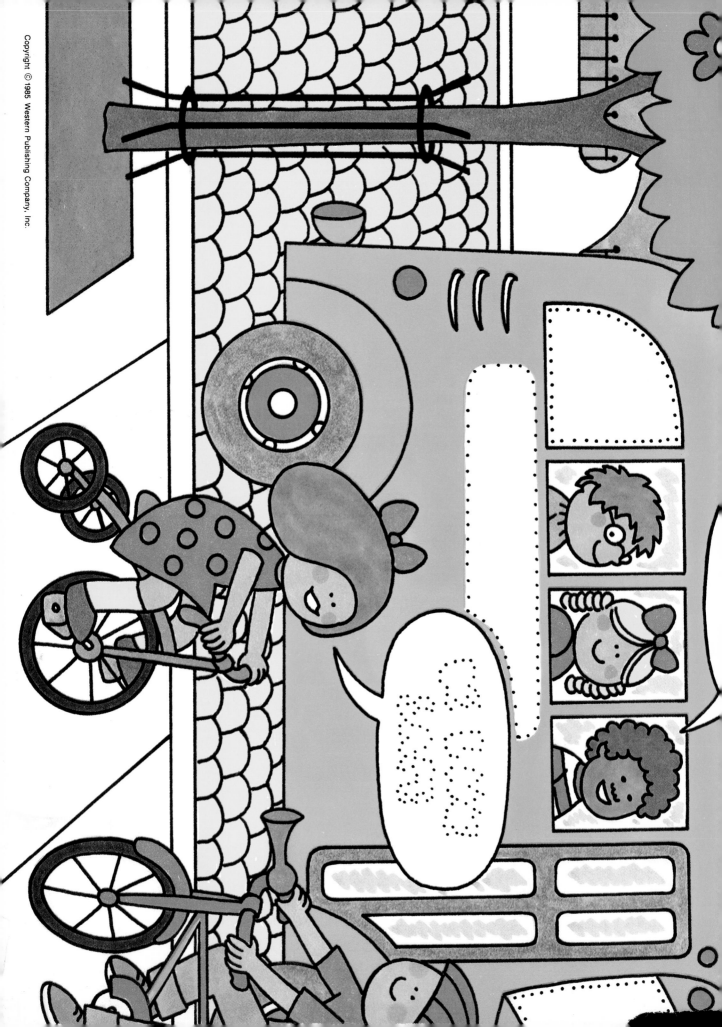

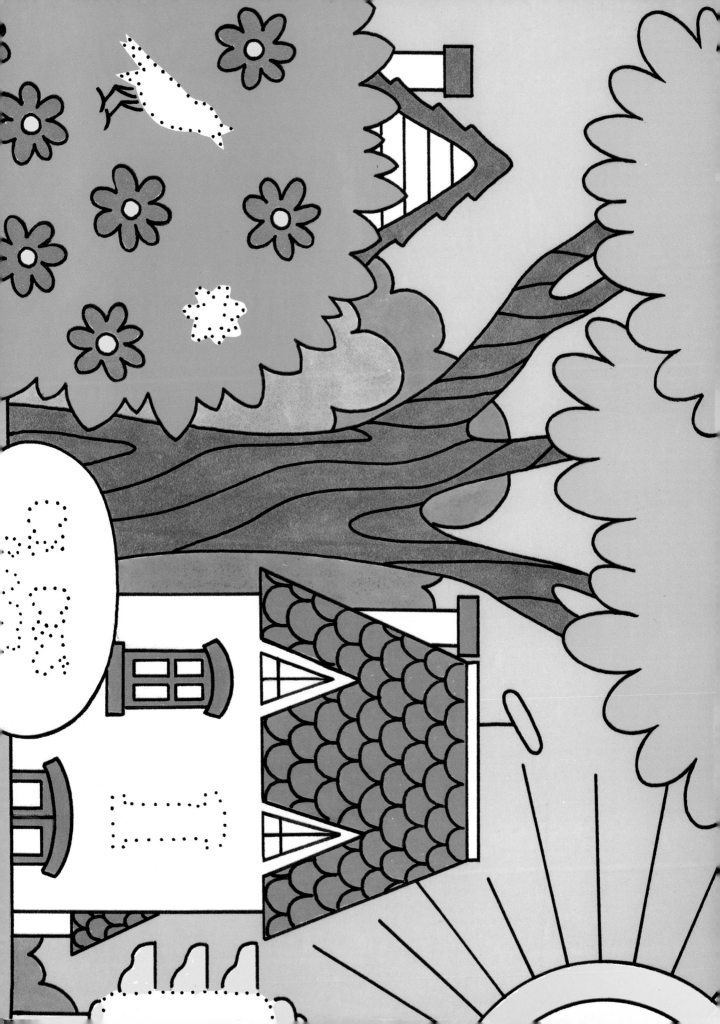

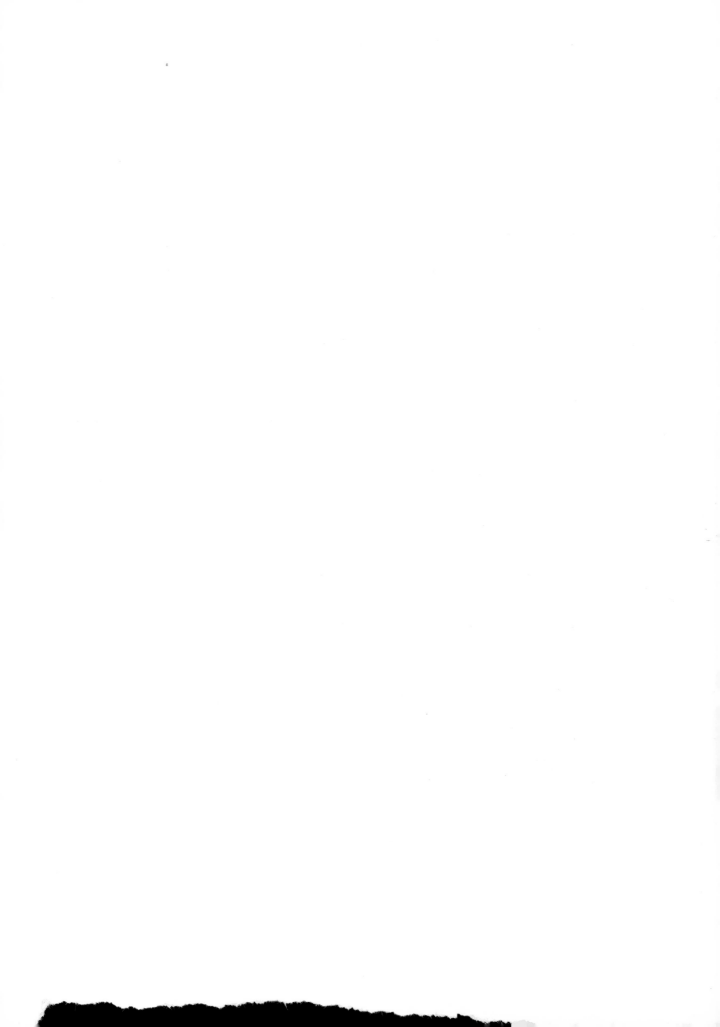

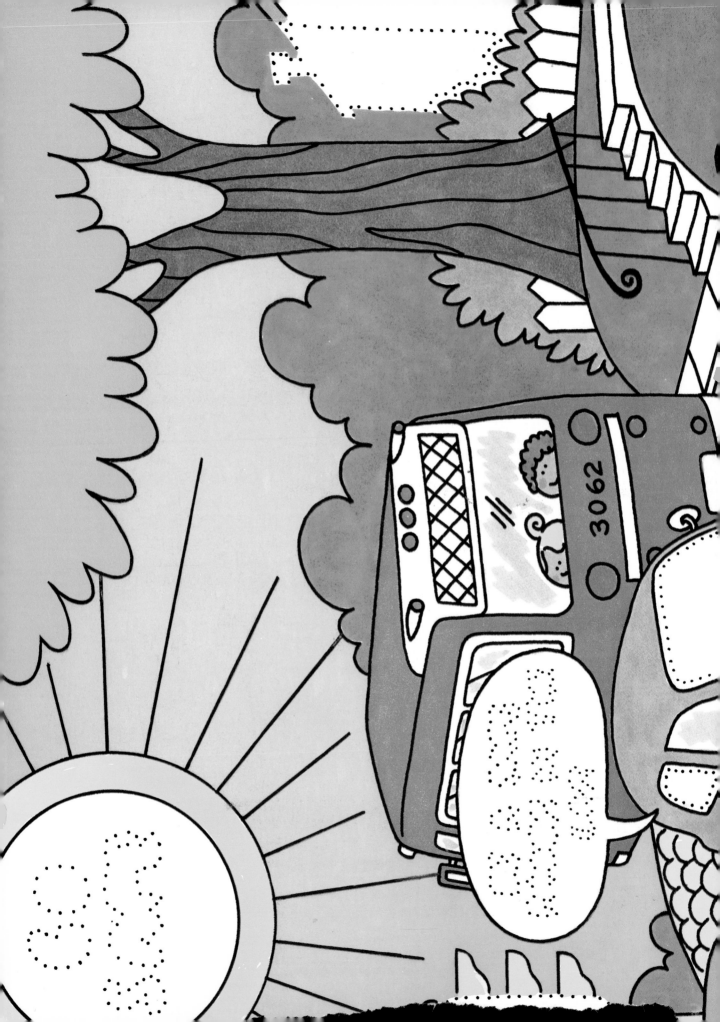

Double Trouble

Bicycles built for one (1) person should have only one (1) person on them (NO RIDERS). Also, carry packages or toys in a basket or a special carrier made for bikes.

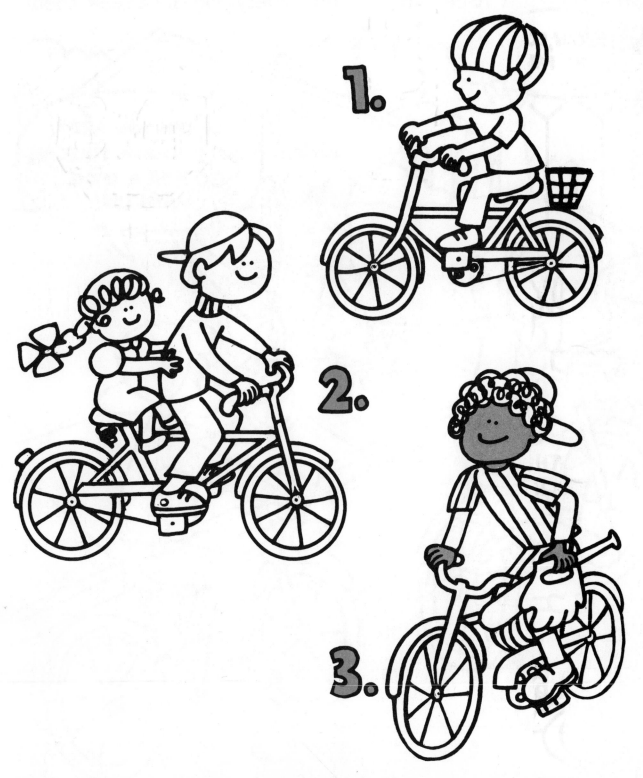

Who is the safe bicycle rider? Draw a circle around the right one.

Obey the Rules

A child under the age of 8 should <u>never</u> ride his or her bicycle on the street. Most communities have rules that deal with safe bicycle riding. Ask your mom or dad to find out what they are. Rules are for your safety. Do not break them!

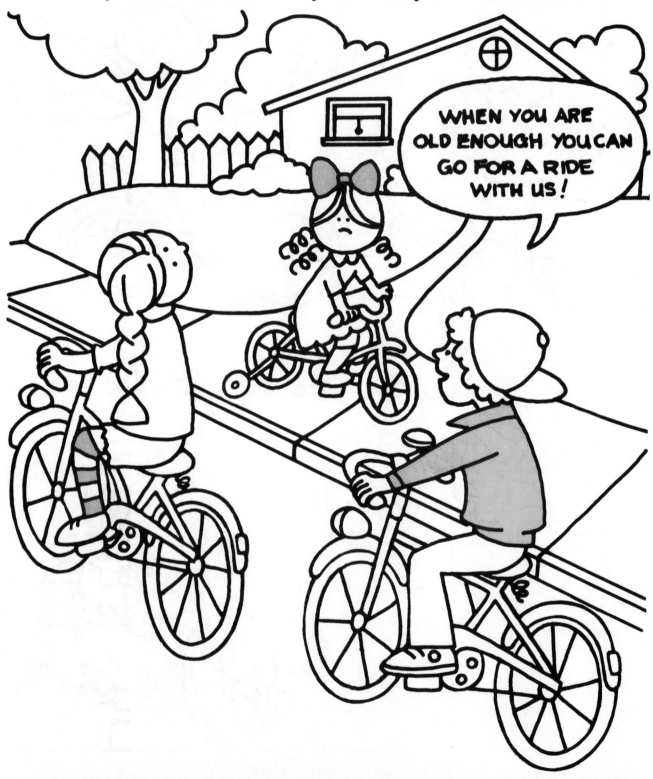

Rules for Older Bike Riders

Children who ride their bicycles on the street should know and follow these important rules. Even though you are not old enough, you can practice them too, while riding on sidewalks or in your own backyard.

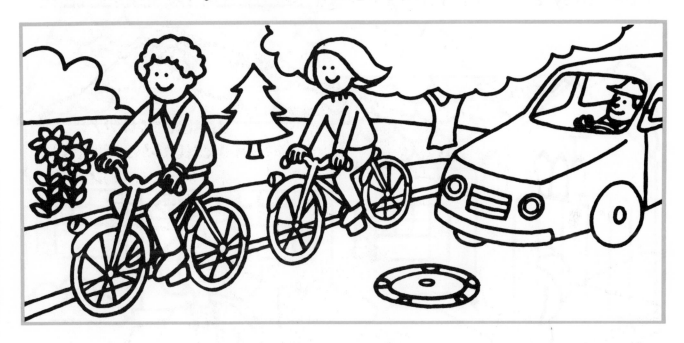

Ride with Traffic

Ride in the same direction as traffic on the right side of the street. Always ride single file.

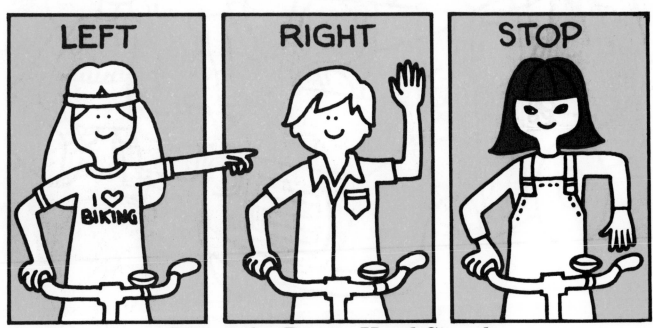

Learn the Proper Hand Signals

Use these hand signals when turning or stopping.

Be Car Safe

This family is going on a trip. Finish the picture so the car will be ready to go.

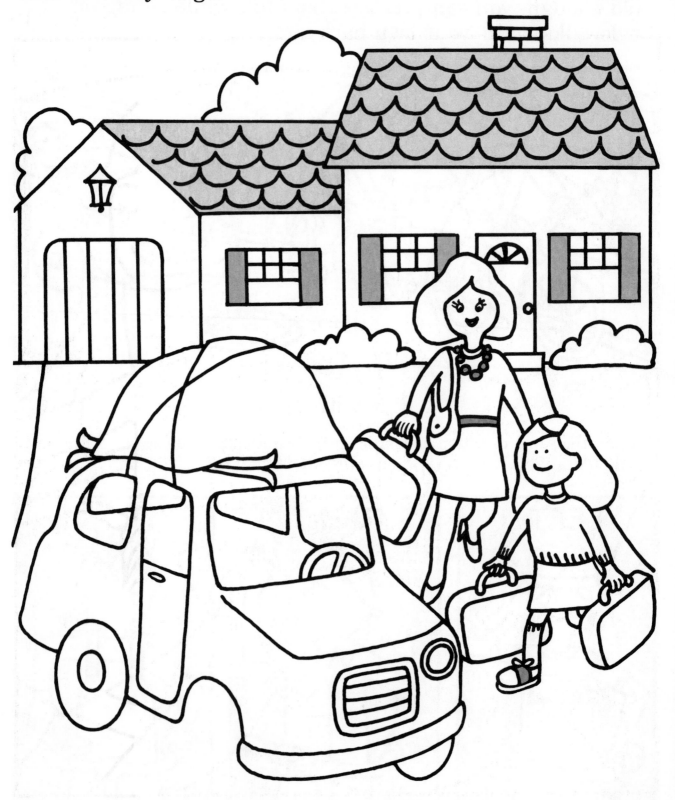

Buckle Up

When everyone is seated, fasten seat belts for safety.
They keep you in place and protect you in case of an accident.

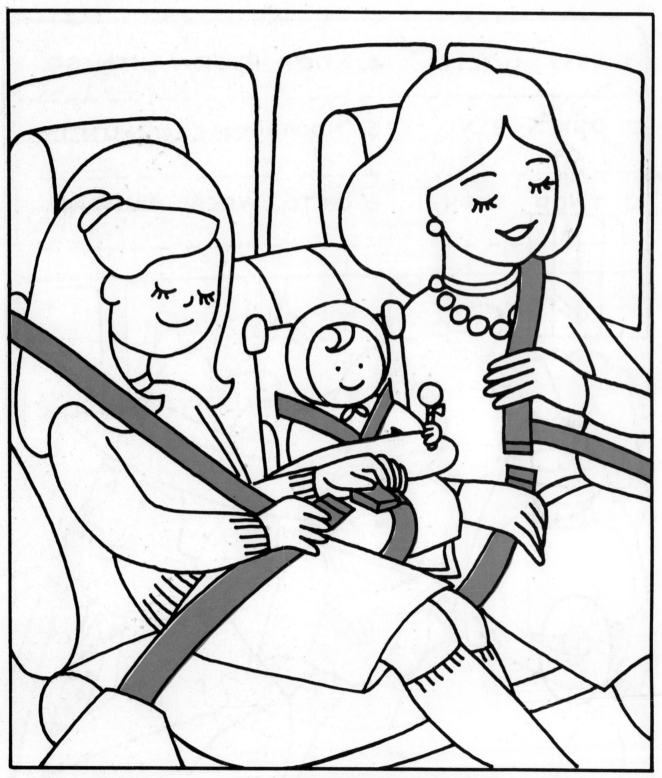

Do you wear your seat belt? Give yourself a reward sticker if you do.

You Can Help the Driver

Here is a list of things you can do to help the driver and have a safer ride. The letters got scrambled. Unscramble them and make the list complete.

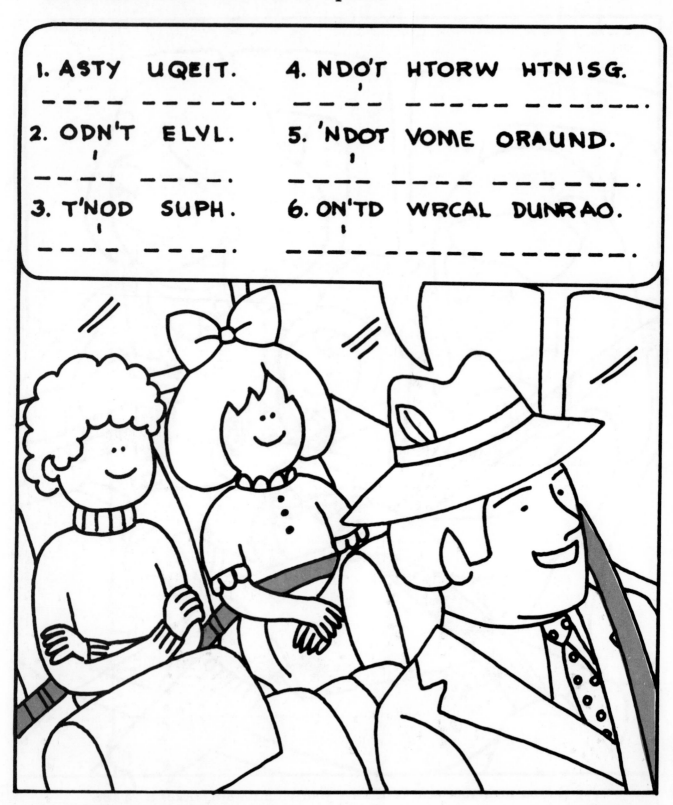

1. ASTY UQEIT.
_____ _____.

2. ODN'T ELVL.
_____ _____.

3. T'NOD SUPH.
_____ _____.

4. NDO'T HTORW HTNISG.
_____ _____ _____.

5. 'NDOT VOME ORAUND.
_____ _____ _____.

6. ON'TD WRCAL DUNRAO.
_____ _____ _____.

State Plates

See how many different states you can find on license plates. Write them down.

Alphabet Fun

Who can be the first one to find all of the letters of the alphabet using street signs and billboards? You can use only one letter from each sign. Each person or team is assigned one side of the street or highway.

Animal Find

Look for animals. See how many different ones you can find.

Be Bus Safe

Here comes the school bus. Do you ride a school bus? Do you know anyone who does? Help take this bus safely to school.

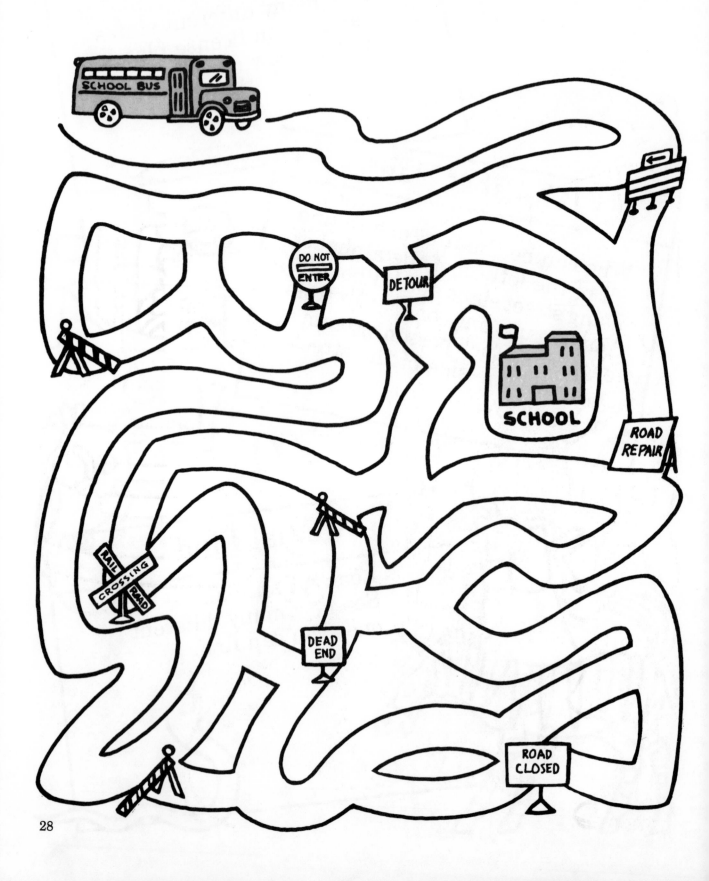

28

Stand in Line

When waiting for the bus, stay out of the road, away from traffic. Don't wander off. If possible, stand with other children who are waiting for the bus, too.

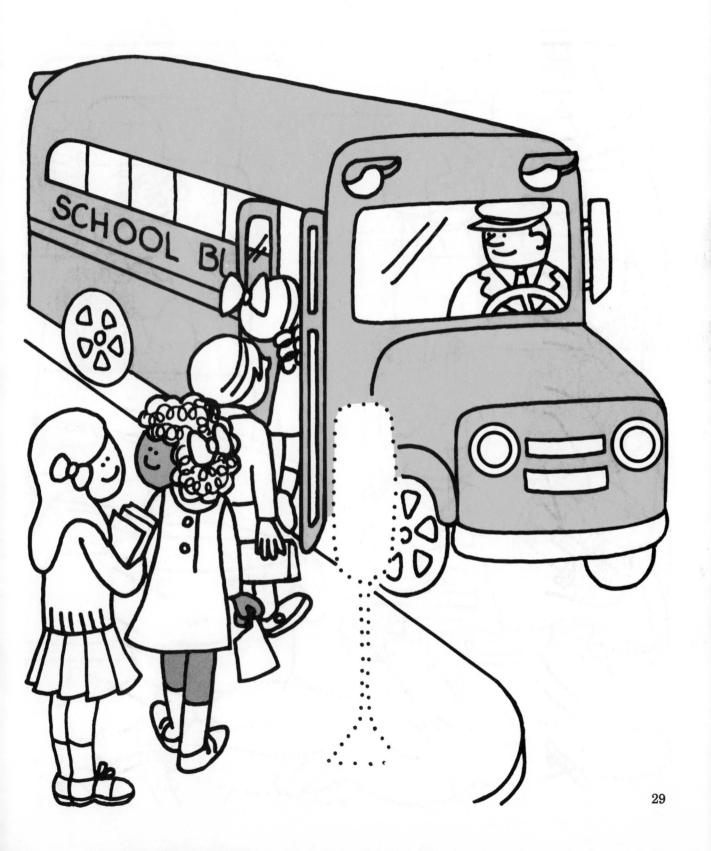

Sitting Still

Find your seat and sit there. It helps the driver do his or her job better when all of the children are sitting down in their seats.

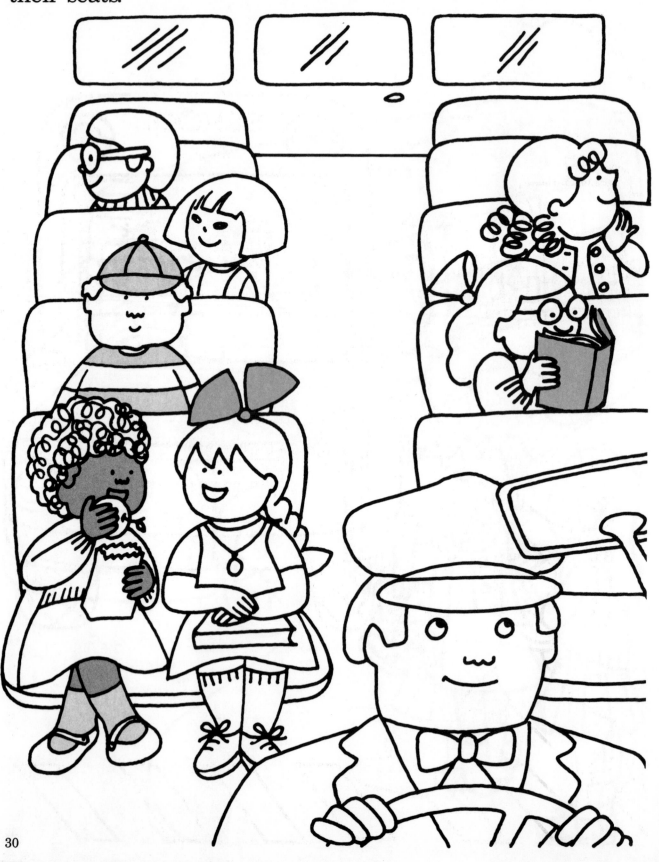

Obey the School Bus Driver

If you must cross the street to get on or off the bus, watch and wait for the driver to motion you across. He or she knows when the path is clear and safe.

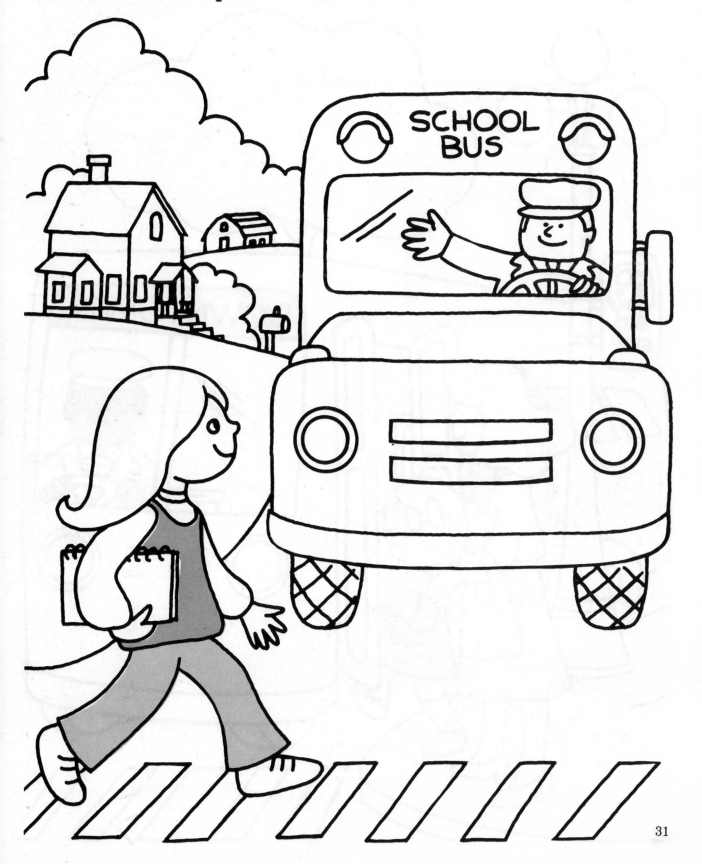

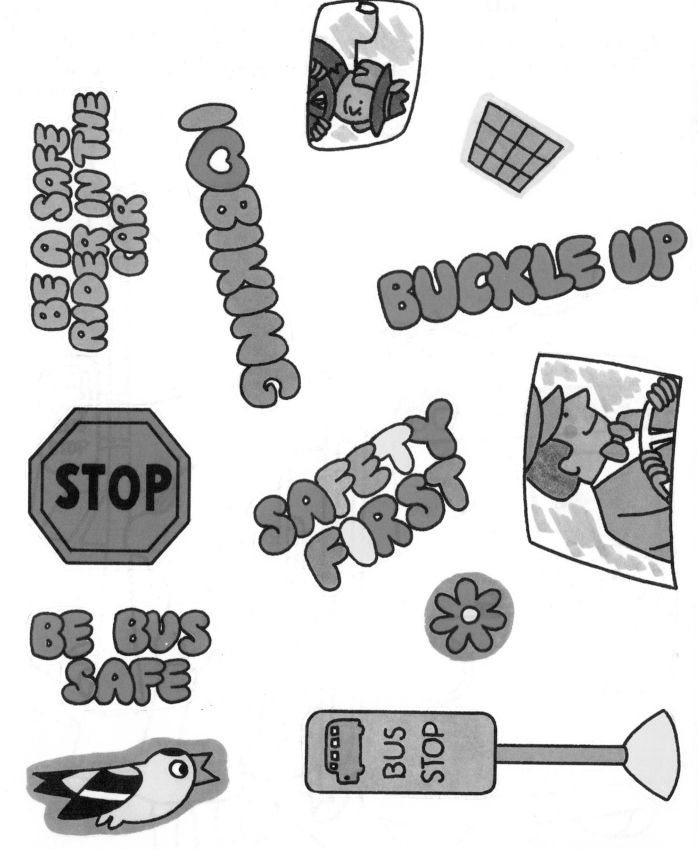